Top 10 Things I Wish Someone Told Me After My Concussions

Lessons learned from a lifetime
of mild TBI recovery

by
BrokenBrilliant

ISBN: 978-1-387-51546-2

For more information on the author and successful brain injury recovery, visit **http://brokenbrilliant.wordpress.com**

This books is for all the
brain injury survivors who are losing hope...
for everyone who has ever been impacted by
concussion and persisting symptoms...
and for all those who persevere

Contents

I HAD A CONCUSSION... NOW WHAT?

When you hit your head hard enough to alter your consciousness, things happen inside your skull that you can't see, but that can affect you in a big way. Medical imaging (MRI, CAT scan, PET scan) can't always pick up the microscopic changes that happen in your brain, but you may notice a lot of subtle changes in how you think, how you move, how you sense the world around you.

Life after concussion (a mild traumatic brain injury, or TBI) can definitely be interesting. And there are lots of lessons to learn. I've had plenty of opportunity to learn those lessons. I've had at least 9 concussions (that I remember - there may have been more), and I'm happy to report that according to most people, I'm "fully recovered". They can't tell any difference between me and how everyone else in the world is.

Inside my head, it's a different story, but I've learned enough over the years, to get me on a positive, pro-active track that's led to living a full and fulfilling life, regardless of my prior injuries. I've learned a lot, and the successful results are obvious to all.

But it took me years to learn a lot of these lessons. Nobody thought to tell me. And the people who knew them, either didn't tell me right away, or weren't available to me when I needed them most.

Here are the top 10 lessons I needed to know, but had to learn the hard way:

1. **You've had a brain injury.** Not once, when I was concussed, did anyone ever tell me that I had a brain injury. Not when I fell, or got hit, or got tackled, or was in a car accident. The idea that my brain was injured -- and I had to take appropriate precautions -- never came up. That may be because the idea of brain injury frightens people. They think of brain damage, and that makes them think of stupidity, idiocy, being "retarded". There's a lot of stigma around brain damage, so brain injury awareness takes a hit, as well. But if I'd know that my brain was injured, that could have made a difference in how I treated myself. I've known for over 30 years that the brain changes -- I just needed to know that I needed to take appropriate action to heal. But I didn't know. So, I didn't do what was necessary.

2. **When the brain is injured, it can release a lot of chemicals that do strange things to the connections that help you think.** The connections that help your brain think may have gotten disconnected and information isn't getting to the right places — like when

electrical wires are frayed and not enough electricity gets through. Just like the lights get dim when there's a brown-out, your brain is having its own brown-out. There may also be a lot of "gunk" in your brain that needs to be cleared out, so that your connections can heal and be repaired.

3. **Your brain has changed.** The connections that used to get information from one place to the next have changed, and your noggin isn't processing things as fast as it used to.

4. **Your ability to plan and follow through may be affected** — you may find pieces of information missing, here and there, and you may not pick up on every detail that you need to make the right decisions.

5. **You are probably going to be more distracted than usual.** Your brain will get confused and not always know what details it should be paying attention to, or remembering. As a result, you might have more trouble remembering things — especially important things, like dates and schedules and appointments.

6. **All of this is going to make you feel very, very tired.** You may need to sleep more than usual. Sleep also helps your brain clear out the gunk that gets released when it gets injured.

7. **Being tired makes you cranky.** It also can make you more emotional than usual. You may find yourself behaving in "strange" ways, or thinking "strange" things. You may also find yourself getting much angrier than before — and much more quickly than before.

8. **You might feel like you are crazy...** like you're losing your mind. You're not. Your brain is just "recalibrating" and figuring out how to do the things it used to do so easily.

9. **You may feel like this for a while.** The best thing you can do is be patient with yourself and be aware of the ways that you are not functioning as well as you would like. Don't rush it. These things take time. Eat healthy food, stay away from a lot of junk food, sugar, caffeine, and stress, drink plenty of water, and get lots of good sleep.

10. **Plenty of other people have had brain injuries / concussions, and most of them**

are getting on with their lives. You may notice some changes in your personality and abilities, but some of the changes may be for the better. Be patient. Pay attention. Be the best person you can. This is not the end.

1. You've Had A Brain Injury.

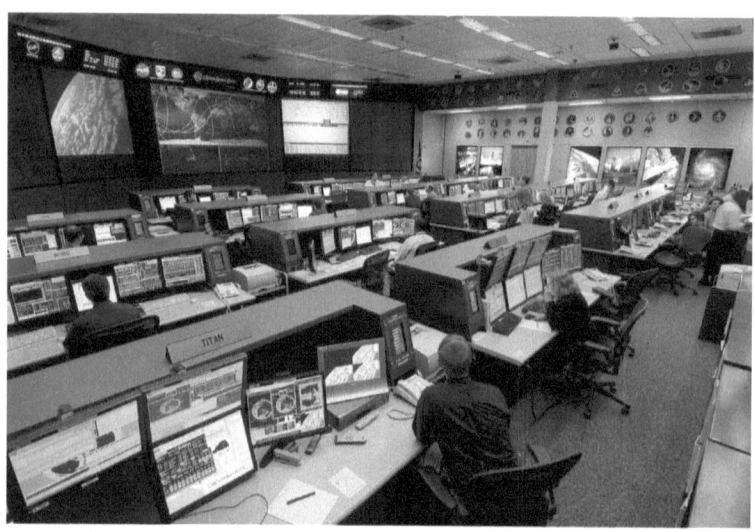

There's a lot going on in "command central"

A concussion is a brain injury.

A mild TBI is a brain injury.

You don't need to get knocked out. You don't need to have amnesia. If you get dazed for even a few seconds, your brain can be injured. It's very simple and very complicated at the same time.

Our brain is "command central"of our bodies and and minds, and an injury to the brain can affect physical systems, as well as mental ones. Vision, balance, hearing, coordination, taste, touch, pain sensations, digestion, sleep/wake cycles... and more... can be screwed up by a brain injury.

So, it's not just about what's in your head – it's about everything that's connected to your brain... your whole body and whole experience as a living, breathing human being can get messed up after a concussion / brain injury.

Even a "mild" TBI can do some serious damage, if you don't treat it properly from the start. If you don't take time to rest and you put extra stress and strain on your system, your body and brain may not have enough time to heal, and you can end up like me – with a lot of personal and professional problems that you have to sort out later.

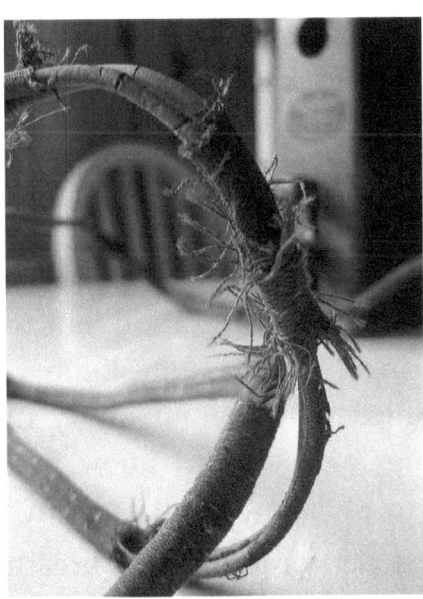

Things get a little frayed...

The connections that help your brain think and messages to the rest of your body may have gotten disconnected and necessary information isn't getting to the right places. Think of what happens when electrical wires get frayed and don't let enough electricity through. The toaster starts making funny noises. The vacuum cleaner just stops for no reason. The cable to your smartphone starts making sputtering noises when you're charging.

Just like the lights get dim when there's a brown-out, your brain is having its own brown-out.

What to do?

Stop. Just stop. You may feel like you need to keep going at top speed, or you're driven to go-go-go, but your brain has been injured, and you need to give it a break. This is serious business, and you need to take a pause and take good care of yourself.

People around you may claim you're "faking it" or you're just trying to get attention, but that says more about them than you. If you skimp on recovering from your concussion / brain injury now, you may end up paying for it later. I know from experience what it's like to pay later, and it's no fun.

Do yourself a favor and take a breather. Just stop. Rest. On the next page you'll find out why.

2. When The Brain Is Injured, It Can Release A Lot Of Chemicals That Do Strange Things To The Connections That Help You Think.

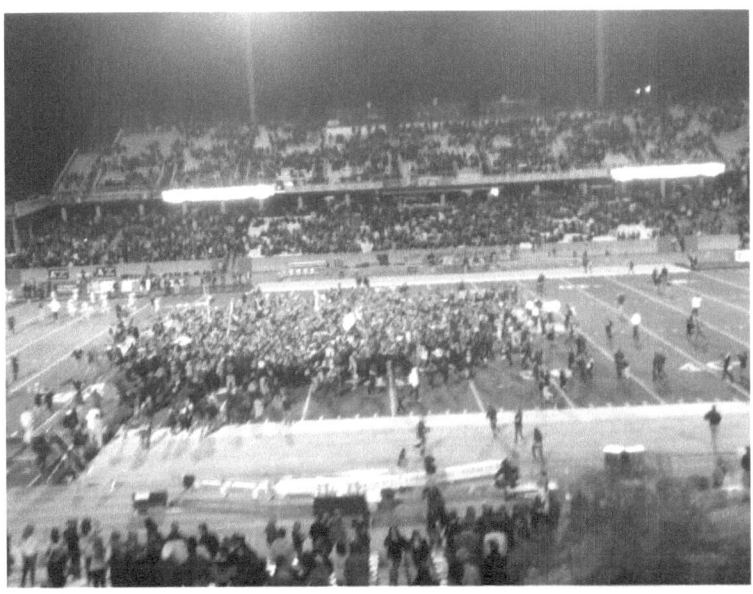

Everybody up and out there! GO-GO-GO!!!

Concussion / mild TBI causes the brain to go hyperactive. It's been injured, and it starts sending out all sorts of messages to the cells without any particular order. It "knows" it's been injured, and it starts telling itself it needs to Get Going! Go! Go! GO!

It's like a commander in war, or a coach in a critical game shouting at the team. The cells themselves start firing on all cylinders – in any and every direction – like soldiers pinned down and desperate to fight their way to safety, firing their guns in all directions with no thought of who or what they might hit. The panicked cells start sending out impulses and communications to each other in no particular order.

In the process, a lot of chemicals that should really stay inside cells, get on the outside. And a lot of chemicals that should stay on the outside, get inside the cells. It's like a panicked football coach telling every single player to get on the field for a play – offense, defense, special teams, and even the kicker, athletic trainers, and support staff end up on the field, running in all directions, none of them quite sure what's supposed to happen, or what they're supposed to do.

All they know is, the coach is yelling GO! GO! GO! ... and they're going.

Scientists call this process a "neurometabolic cascade" -- a chain reaction that releases all sorts of interesting biochemical substances into places of the brain that normally shouldn't have them there. Cell walls get "breached" and the stuff that used to be inside gets outside, and the stuff that used to be outside gets inside.

In concussion / mild TBI, your brain is literally flooded with chemicals that shouldn't be where they are. If you've ever had your basement flooded, or you've seen pictures of a flood aftermath, you get the general idea of what happens to the brain.

Even after the initial excitation is over, it takes a while for the brain's processes to return to normal. Just like a flood leaves a coating of gunk behind it, all the chemicals in the wrong places leave gunk on the connections in your brain.

Depending on the concussion, there may be a lot of "gunk" that your brain needs to clear out before its connections can begin to heal and be repaired.

During that time – sometimes it's days, sometimes weeks, sometimes months (it varies from person to person) – your brain has to work extra overtime to clean up its act. The problem is, it takes extra energy for it to do that – and the metabolic energy-producing process involved is negatively affected by concussion.

So, just at the time when the brain needs more energy to clean out and heal, it's less able to produce the energy it needs.

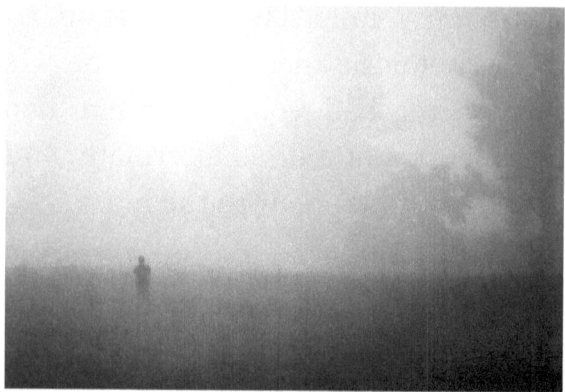

Feels like a fog - 'cause it is

The net result? You may feel like you're walking around in a fog. And you are.

Your brain's connections are "fogged up" by the extra gunk that got released when you got "dinged". It's a terrible feeling – especially if you're the kind of person who's always on the go, always active and involved in life. If you "just bumped your head", it might not make any sense to feel the way you do – but you feel this way for a very good reason: your brain is still trying to clean itself out, so it can get on with the healing process.

You're not stupid – it just feels that way. And chances are good that you won't feel that way forever.

Think of what happens when water gets in your gas tank. The engine doesn't much like it, and it lets you know. It sputters and coughs and can sound like it has a nasty cold. Likewise, when all those neurochemicals clog up your system after a brain injury, the engine inside your head starts to behave strangely, too.

Depending on your injury, some of the connections themselves might actually be frayed or broken... but you won't be able to tell, until after the neurochemical gunk has been cleared away.

What to do?

Sleep, clean drinking water, and nutritious food have all been shown to help.

Some people take supplements like fish oil to help, but some people (like me) have reactions to it, so it's really best to keep things super-simple.

Just resting and taking a break from all the screens, and not doing a lot of mental activity are highly recommended. T.V., reading, video games, Facebook, surfing the web, emailing... all those things get your brain riled up, so you need to step away from them for a while, so your brain can catch up with itself.

Sleeping is actually one of the best things you can do for yourself, because it's been shown to help clear out gunk from the brain. While we are asleep, the brain is literally washing itself, so one of the smartest things you can do after a concussion is give it plenty of opportunity to do the work for you.

Trust me, it's no fun. Your brain is telling itself (and your body) to Go-Go-Go, but remember, it's been injured, and it has no idea what you're supposed to do. That's just the neurotransmitters talking.

3. Your Brain Has Changed.

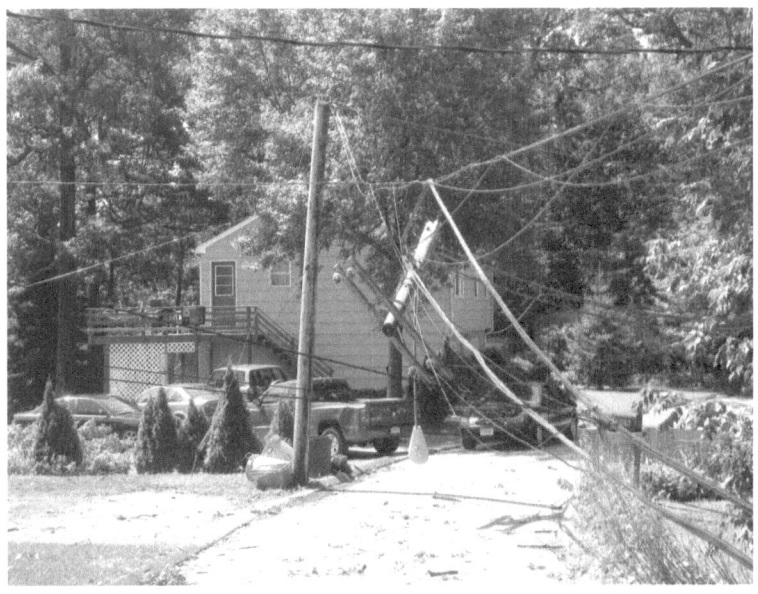

It's like this

Concussion changes the brain.

First, it floods it with chemicals that aren't supposed to be where they go. And sometimes those chemicals can actually damage healthy cells.

The connections that used to get information from one place to the next can be altered.

Depending on the type of concussion, there can be bleeding, twisting, or shearing of connections, that make it harder for information to get where it needs to go.

Concussion is like a microburst that suddenly appears in a normally quiet neighborhood, blowing out windows, uprooting shrubbery and trees, pulling down power and cable lines, tossing lawn furniture into the street, and seriously rearranging the garbage cans that were neatly lined along the driveway. Even a quick hit or a "ding" can do some real damage.

Clearing out the gunk that gets loose in your brain is a lot like clearing the wreckage after a microburst. First you have to pick up all the loose trash, then you have cut apart the trees that pulled down the power lines. Only after you get the big trees out and stand up the poles, can you tell if the electricity and phone lines are still any good.

Maybe some of them are fine.

Maybe others got pulled out of their connections, and utility crews need to just tighten them up.

And maybe some of the wires got so frayed and torn that they need to be replaced. That replacement takes time. New crews need to be called in. Maybe a crew isn't available, or they don't have the needed parts. The neighborhood is going to be out of power and cable for a bit.

That's basically how it is after a concussion / TBI. Sometimes that proverbial microburst does damage to the actual connections in your brain.

And if you've had a prior concussion (or two or three – or nine, like me), your brain can have an even harder time getting information from one place to the next.

Imagine a neighborhood that's had a lot of storms that knocked out power. Utilities crews have patched up the connections many, many times – and each time the connection gets a little easier to damage, because all the loosening and tightening and adjusting puts a strain on the materials used. Screws get stripped. Casings on cables get thin. Wires get twisted and re-twisted, weakening them in the process. Connectors get overloaded with additional cables. And while the system does restart, with each new storm, the power goes out that much more easily.

Repeat concussions are pretty much like that.

Connections in the brain aren't the only thing that can suffer after getting your bell rung.

When the information crosses the wires and actually gets where it's going, the "microprocessors" that used to figure out what to do with it may have altered.

Our brains are incredibly complex, and they process billions upon billions of pieces of data on a moment-by-moment basis. When our neurochemical process is messed up, it can make it harder to figure out what to do with the information that comes through over our stressed "wiring".

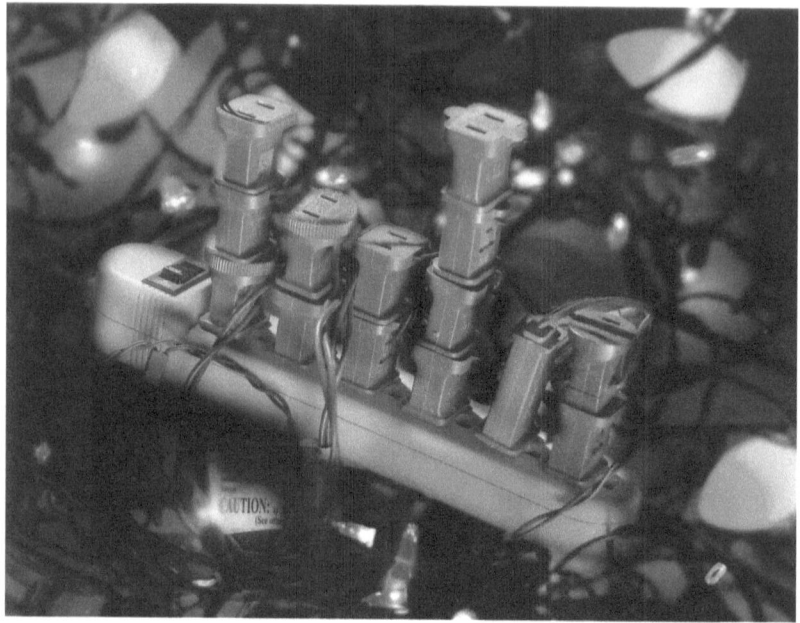

There's too much input and activity for our systems to take at one time

Let's go back to that neighborhood that got hit by the microburst.

When the utility crews finally have the electricity back on, and cable is restored, can life go back to normal immediately?

Not if everyone in the neighborhood is exhausted from the cleanup. Even if you do have electricity and cable, surfing the channels is going to be a challenge, if you're wiped out from all the hauling and cutting and cleanup efforts. You'll have cable back, but when you use the remote, you fingers will hit the wrong buttons and you might have trouble reading the listings on your t.v. screen. If you're getting on Facebook, you might have trouble typing or understanding what others have posted, because you're so tired.

Even though you have electricity and cable, you still have trouble using them.

And that's how it can be in your brain after concussion. Even if the information is getting through from synapse to synapse, once it gets there, the synapses may not know how to handle the info correctly.

As a result, your noggin isn't processing things the way it used to.

It can feel a lot sssssllllllooooooowwwwwerrrrrrrr.

You can feel like life is moving in slow motion.

And in a way, it is. Because the thing that observes and interprets your life is not firing on all cylinders. Not yet, anyway.

You can feel like you're walking around in a fog. And you are. Remember the "gunk" that got released in your brain? It takes a while to clear it out, and in the meantime, your brain is struggling to connect the dots in your daily life – with connections that don't work like they used to.

What to do?

Again, getting plenty of sleep, water, and nutritious food are really good for you.

Probably the most important thing is to avoid stress.

Stress is a killer. It limits the brain's ability to learn – which is exactly what it needs to do after a concussion / TBI. Stress can put you in fight-flight mode that makes you aggressive and combative – which can get you into even more trouble with people like the authorities or other people who just want to fight.

Whatever you do for yourself after concussion, you've got to take it easy on yourself and give yourself plenty of time to get back. You can get back. Lots of people have gotten injured like you, and the majority of them have returned to their regular lives. TBI and concussion are extremely common, so rest assured you're in good company.

Unfortunately, stress goes hand-in-hand with TBI and concussion. I can't tell you how to stop the stress, but I can tell you how to limit the negative effects.

Deep Relaxation has been unbelievably helpful for me, over the past years. For a long, long time, I had no interest in relaxation. I hated to relax, in fact. Turns out, I just didn't know how. But I found a recording for progressive relaxation that I could listen to, and it helped me train myself to let go of all the stress and feel normal again.

You might not be able to stop the stresses of life, but you can stop the negative effect it has on you.

Take your injury seriously and give yourself time to recover. And learn to offset the stress to your system with rest and relaxation.

4. Your Ability To Plan And Follow Through May Be Affected, And You Might Not Be Able To Make Good Judgments.

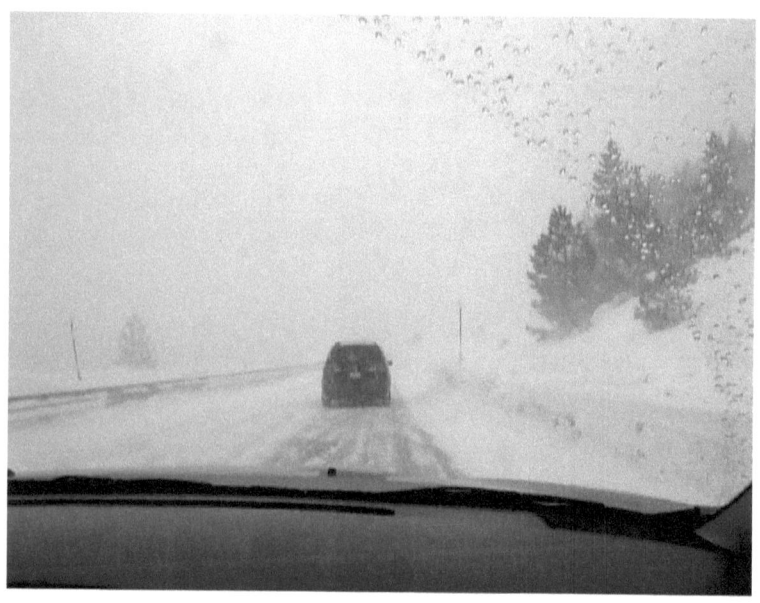

You may think it's safe to drive... when it's not

One of the worst things about TBI is that it can hide itself very well from the very people who are having trouble. An injured brain doesn't always know it's injured, and it usually wants to jump back in the action before it's ready.

But it doesn't know it's not ready, because it can't tell that it's injured.

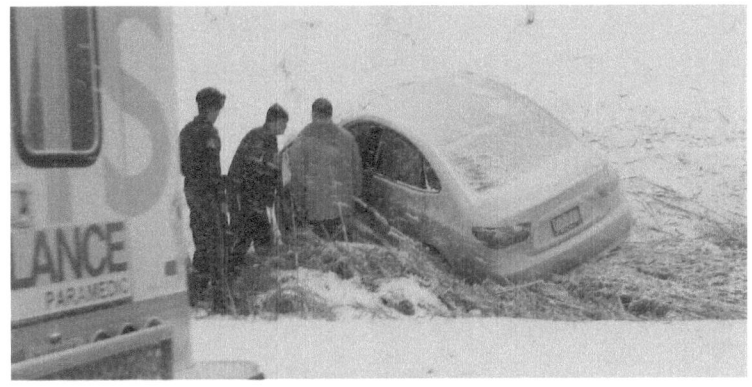

... And then this happens

If you remember nothing else, at least remember this:

After concussion, your brain will usually over-estimate your ability to do regular things again. And it will often tell you that you can do things even better than before... but you can't.

I wish someone had told me about this danger after so many of my concussions.

Of course, even if they had, I probably wouldn't have believed them. I interviewed for jobs that were far, far above my professional grade. Somehow, I was convinced that if another person could do the job of a C-level executive, I could, too. I told interviewers that I was capable of becoming an executive at companies where I had little to no experience because, "If they can do it, so can I."

If you think I got a lot of strange looks at job interviews... you're right.

I also had many close calls after making poor judgments around people carrying guns.

I nearly got myself killed while walking down a deer path in the early morning hours during deer hunting season, wearing no bright colors, and actually wanting to blend in like deer, so I could catch sight of one. I was nearly shot by a hunter, who pulled up before he pulled the trigger.

I also got into numerous scrapes with police officers, because I misunderstood what they were saying to me, and I got aggressive in response. I've resisted arrest, went out of my way to get confrontational with armed officers, and I've barely escaped a number of close calls with jail, thanks to lack of impulse control and terrible judgment – thanks to all those TBIs I've sustained.

And that's just scratching the surface. I can tell you from plenty of personal experience that brain injury screws with your ability to think clearly and make good decisions.

This is to be expected. It's completely normal for people who sustain concussions / TBIs.

Planning and good decision-making are some of the top casualties in brain injury, for a number of reasons:

A) You're not getting all the info you need to make good choices.

B) The thinking process that decides what's good or bad may be impaired.

C) You might not have the energy or patience to sort through all the details and come up with a good plan.

D) Your impulse control might not be great, so you jump into things before you think them through.

E) You may be extremely anxious, which makes you do things too quickly – or not at all.

There are plenty more reasons, but these are the Big Five that cause many problems.

Basically, you may find pieces of information missing, here and there... or you may not pick up on every detail that you need to make the right decisions.

It's kind of like a contestant in a beauty pageant who has a salad for lunch and then is so caught up in thinking about her hair and her dress, that she doesn't check her teeth in the mirror before she goes out for the next round on stage. The camera pans across the line of smiling contestants, and there she is with a big piece of dark green spinach on her teeth.

Not good. Chances are, her shot at the title is gone.

Even if you really, really want to do the right thing in the right way, your brain might not be up to the task of doing it... yet. Here's why:

The frontal lobes – the very front of the brain in your forehead above your eyes – is the part of the brain that helps us plan our lives, follow through, and make wise decisions. And because it's out there in front, it's especially susceptible to injury.

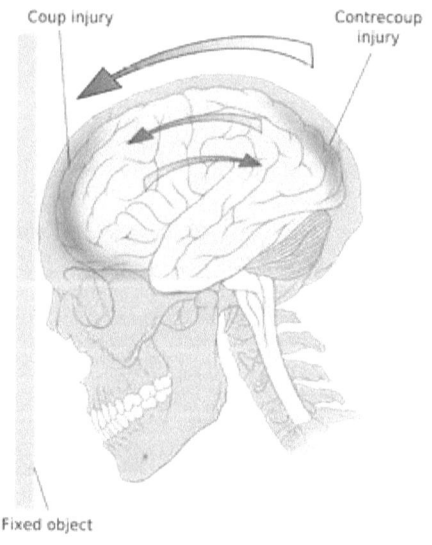

Double-whammy

Even if you get hit in the back of the head – like when you get rear-ended in traffic – your brain can smack up against the inside of the front of your skull. This is not good news for anyone, because the inside of the skull is sharp and bony, and the brain is soft like Jell-O.

When your executive function is impaired, your brain can get you into a ton of really bad scrapes. That includes telling yourself that you're ready to get back into playing, working, or learning long before you're ready to. It also includes telling yourself that you're a lot better at something than you are.

Impaired executive function can go hand-in-hand with impaired risk assessment (where you can't really tell how dangerous a situation is before jumping in), so you can put yourself in real danger without realizing it.

Some examples:

- Getting back into extreme sports when your coordination and timing are not nearly as good as they used to be.
- Starting classes again and taking even harder ones than before, when your brain isn't processing info as well as it once was.
- Taking up a new sport you never played before and trying to jump to expert level participation right away.
- Getting involved with illegal activities.

- Confronting an armed motorist who's caught up in road rage.

These can all get you hurt. They can also get you killed. But if your executive function is impaired, you're not exactly qualified to make those kinds of decisions.

One of the biggest problems with brain injury / concussion is that it also tricks you into thinking that there's no problem at all with your thinking. You're sure that you're fine!

This special brand of confusion is so common that there's even a word for not knowing that you don't know you're impaired: **anosognosia**.

Your brain can be so injured that it's literally incapable of telling how good or bad it is at...well, anything. This is common after stroke, as well as more serious brain injuries.

And it's very, very dangerous. Combine poor judgment with the impatience and anxiety that often comes with TBI, and you have a powder keg just waiting to go off.

It's nobody's fault, and it doesn't mean there's something wrong with you, if you keep making bone-headed mistakes.

It just means that part of your brain that's responsible for "executive functioning" is impaired and needs some help.

What to do?

In many concussions, poor judgment is either temporary or it can be offset by some help from other people or tools you can use.

The most important thing is to understand that your brain can – and will – play tricks on you after a concussion or TBI. It doesn't mean you're permanently damaged, it just means you need to re-train that part of your brain to A) slow down to notice the right details, and B) get in the habit of thinking things through.

If you've got friends to bounce ideas off, this is the best time to use them.

If you don't have friends in the "real world" (they may have ditched you after your injury, or you might be isolated by your problems), you can find online support groups who can help you sort things out.

Also, there are professionals who can help you with your decision-making. You may be able to find a counselor or neuropsychologist who can help you retrain your brain to think more systematically and come up with better solutions to problems.

The best thing you can probably do, is reach out for help. Because your brain is going to tell you some interesting things – many of those things may be 100% wrong... but you'll never know it, because your brain doesn't.

5. You Are Probably Going To Be More Distracted Than Usual.

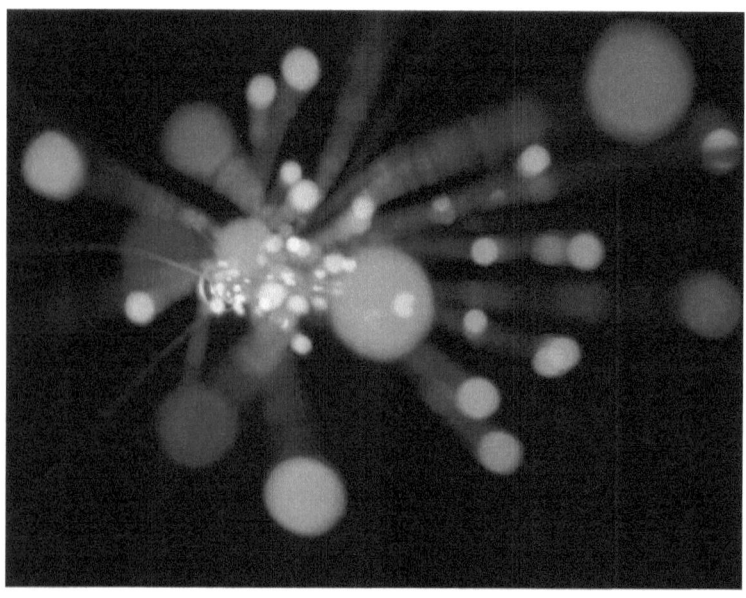

Everything looks important

Brain injury can make people very distractable. In my case, I am very light and noise sensitive, so on bad days, every passing shadow or bright light or sound catches my attention. With all the excitatory neurochemicals loose in our brains after concussion, our brains are on high-alert, and that can make us instantly notice tons of details that don't mean a thing.

Your brain can get confused and not always know what details it should be paying attention to. It can get confused about what it really important and what it can safely ignore.

And because you have so much rattling 'round in your head, you might have more trouble remembering things — especially important things, like dates and schedules and appointments.

It actually takes a lot of brain power to notice lots of details and know what to pay attention to, and it takes special attention to commit things to memory. If your brain is so busy noticing everything and categorizing it without understanding what's really going on, it's not going to have a lot of bandwidth to devote to memorizing critical things.

Concussion / TBI is stressful, and stress make us more distracted than usual. It puts us on "high alert" where we think everything is important and needs to be noticed. This is a huge energy drain, and it tires you out even more.

A tired brain is a distractable brain.

And distraction makes the brain work harder, as it tries to "track" all the different pieces of information and put them in some kind of order – which makes it even more tired.

See the irony?

Yes, you're right. It does suck.

What to do?

Again... sleep. Get plenty of rest. Your brain needs to heal, and pushing the envelope isn't going to help. A tired brain is a distractable brain, so the less tired it is, the better your chances.

There are exercises you can do to increase your focus. Puzzles can help, and some online training supposedly helps, as well.

Meditation and mindfulness are highly recommended. They can literally alter the structure of the brain and strengthen the areas for focus.

Be careful of medication. Some meds actually make the brain more tired (some anti-depressants), which doesn't help with concentration after a brain injury. Other meds will get you cranked up to high speed, which can fry your system. Be careful with meds, even over the counter ones. And talk to your doctor, if you're concerned.

6. All Of This Is Going To Make You Feel Very, *Very* Tired.

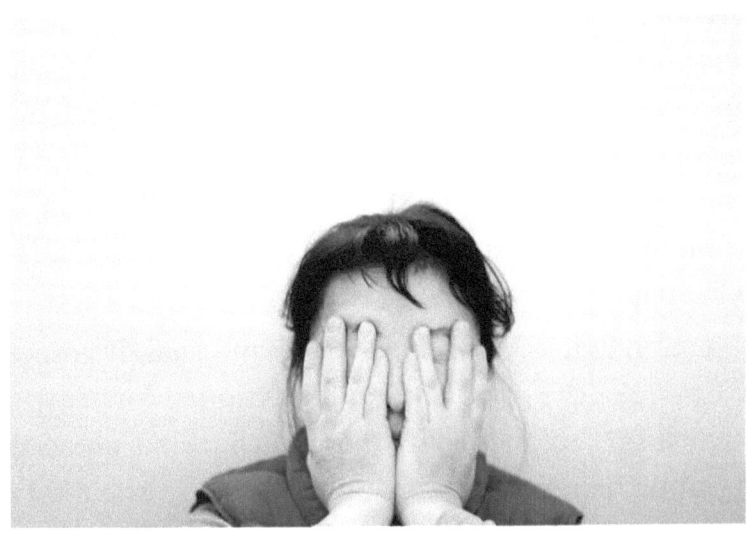

TBI / concussion symptoms can drain you.

The sleep thing again...

I'm repeating myself, because it's that important.

Fatigue is one of the top complaints of people who have sustained a brain injury. For some, it resolves in a matter of weeks or months, for others (myself included), it goes on for years. Giving yourself a chance to heal up front is probably a good idea.

TBI / concussion can make you feel wiped out.

When your brain is going haywire and it's sending strange messages to your body, and your body is hyper-sensitive to just about everything... it's exhausting. I spent years in a near-constant state of exhaustion. I had maybe a few good hours in the morning, then I was done.

Especially at the start, when your brain is figuring everything out – it feels like for the first time – you can end up feeling fried before you get half-way through the day. I drank way too much coffee for years, just to keep going. I didn't understand what the problem was. I just knew I was exhausted, and I had to keep going.

You may need to sleep more than usual. If you can get it – take the opportunity. I functioned for years on exhaustion, because I had no choice. I had no access to public benefits, and if I didn't work, I didn't eat or have a home. So, I worked. Through the exhaustion. It was no fun at all – for me, or for my loved ones. We all paid a steep price for my fatigue.

What to do?

Sleep is precious. It helps your brain clear out the gunk that gets released when it gets injured, and it restores your sanity. Get as much sleep as you can, whenever you can.

You may feel like a loser for needing so much sleep, and/or others might call you a "slacker", but they don't live with your brain. You do. Give it a break. Give yourself a chance to feel human again.

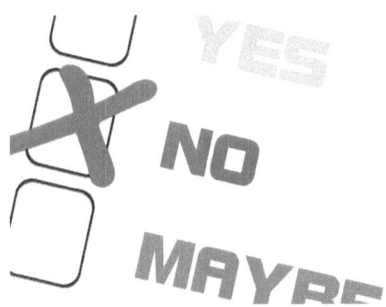

Also, consider cutting back on all the stuff you think you need to do.

A lot of us stay busy, just because everyone else does it, or it makes us feel more productive and needed. In the end, you might be productive and needed, but you still feel like death-warmed-over. It's up to you, but I've found that cutting back on all my customary activities was a magical relief.

All the "friends" I used to have? They're still running on their hamster wheels. And they're no happier now, than when I departed from their midst.

7. Being Tired Makes You Cranky. It Also Can Make You More Emotional Than Usual.

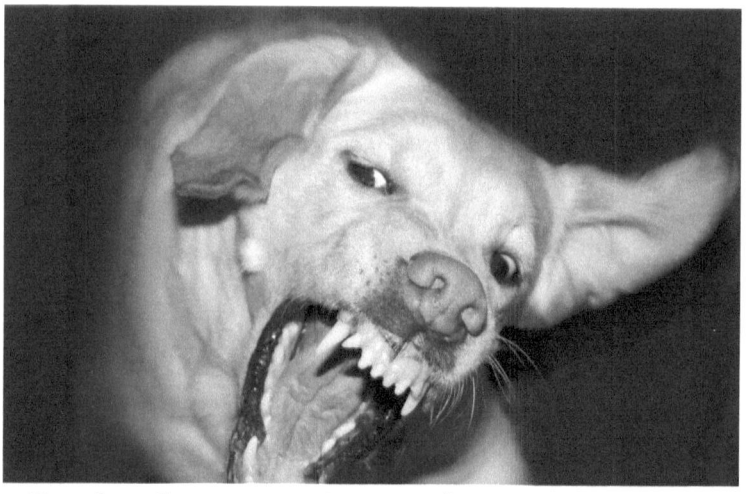

Cranky after concussion? You're not the only one

You may find yourself behaving in "strange" ways, or thinking "strange" things. You may also find yourself getting much angrier than before — and much more quickly than before.

A tired brain isn't just a distractable brain – it's an irritable brain, as well. Fatigue can cause an injured brain to overreact – to everything. It can give you a hair-trigger temper and make you unpredictable and volatile.

That's not good for anyone.

I wish I'd known this from the start. It would have saved me so many years of real pain over watching myself blow up over nothing... at times becoming a danger to myself and the people around me.

I blew up with family, friends, co-workers, bosses, healthcare professionals, and yes, police officers. I lost jobs and relationships because of this.

It was so debilitating to watch myself go ballistic over things like dropping a spoon on the kitchen floor, or not being able to understand what people were saying to me. If I had known what fatigue does to my brain – because of my injuries – I would have worried less about being a bad person, and worried more about getting to bed at a decent hour.

What to do?

Pay attention to how tired you are. And pay attention to when you have a bad day – or a bad incident. Notice any connection?

To combat this problem, you can schedule important things for the morning, when you are still fresh. And you can postpone (or avoid) doing social things when you are tired.

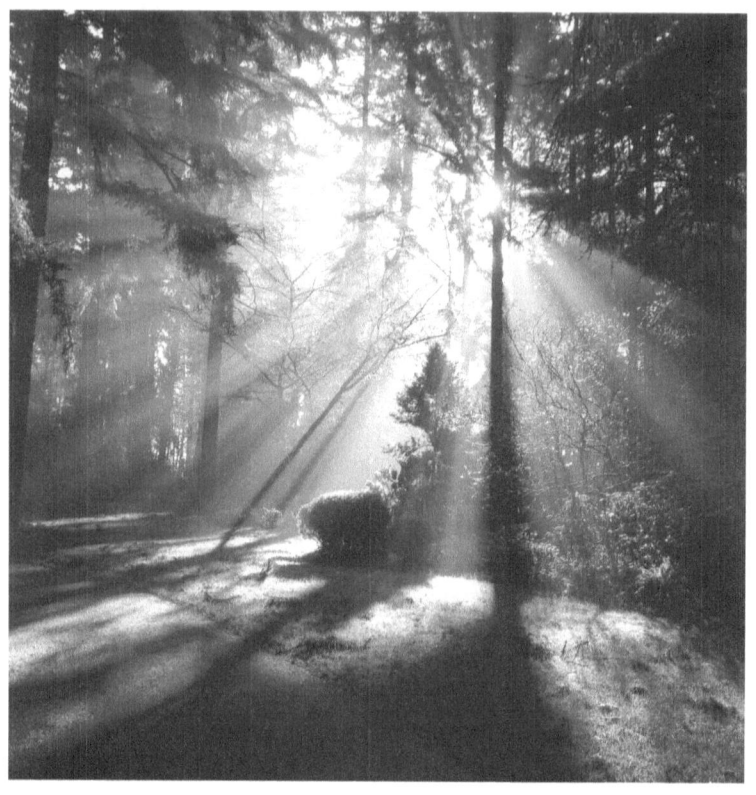

Earlier tends to be better for a lot of us

Important activities where you need to keep your cool need to happen when you're not fatigued. And that means doing important things earlier in the week, too.

By Friday, no matter how early it is in the morning, you may still be tired enough to fly off the handle over nothing at all.

There are medications that can help with the exhaustion that comes with TBI. Some meds will help you think better, so you get less tired, period.

If you want to go "med-less" (that's what I prefer), you can always have a cup of coffee before an important event. But you have to watch out that it's not too late in the day, or it may keep you from getting to sleep. A cup of coffee at 3:45 p.m. may help for that Thursday-afternoon meeting, but it may put the screws to your Friday.

8. You Might Feel Like You Are Crazy... Like You're Losing Your Mind.

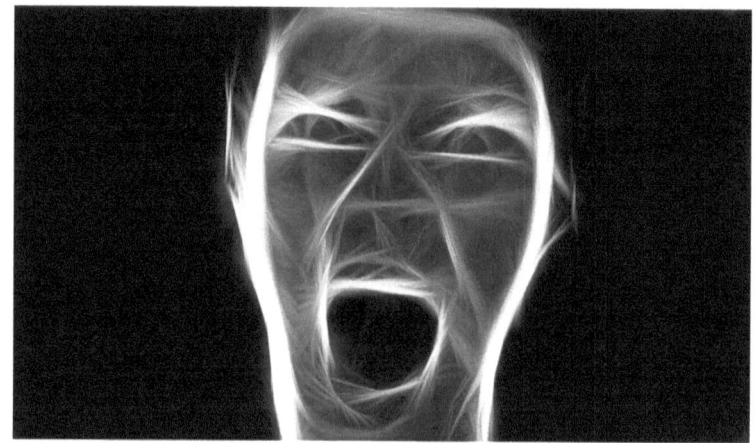

Auuuuggghhhh!

This is another very common complaint after concussion / TBI. Your brain is working differently than before. Maybe you're saying and doing things that don't make sense to you – and others around you. Maybe you can't find the right words. Maybe your body is super-sensitive to every little stimulus. And you certainly don't feel like your old self.

Believe me, this is common. Thousands upon thousands of people with concussion / TBI feel like they're losing their minds. Some feel that way longer than others, but for the vast majority, they get back to feeling normal before too long.

That's how it was for me for many years. I'd get hit on the head, be dazed and confused for some time... then eventually I'd be back to feeling like myself. This last time, it took me 10 years to start feeling like myself again. But at least I'm back. For the most part.

Some days, I still feel like a stranger. And I don't know what happened to the old me I used to know so well.

Yes, it can make you feel crazy.

But you're not crazy. Your brain is just "recalibrating" and figuring out how to do the things it used to do so easily.

It's not a small thing, however. This complicates life in so many ways – including your interactions with others. One way it is particularly troublesome, is with doctors. If you have trouble expressing yourself and words aren't coming out properly, it can be hard, if not impossible, to get good medical help. In my case, I was so "all over the map" that one neurologist after another treated me like I was mentally ill and just looking for attention and pills. Needless to say, it made it hard to get help. But I stuck with it, and my persistence paid off.

Unfortunately, not everyone is as fortunate as I have been.

The important thing to remember – no matter what doctors or friends or family members say – is that the source of your troubles is your brain. It's not something you're making up. It's real. And you need to reckon with it.

Remember that neighborhood I talked about earlier? The one that got hit with the microburst?

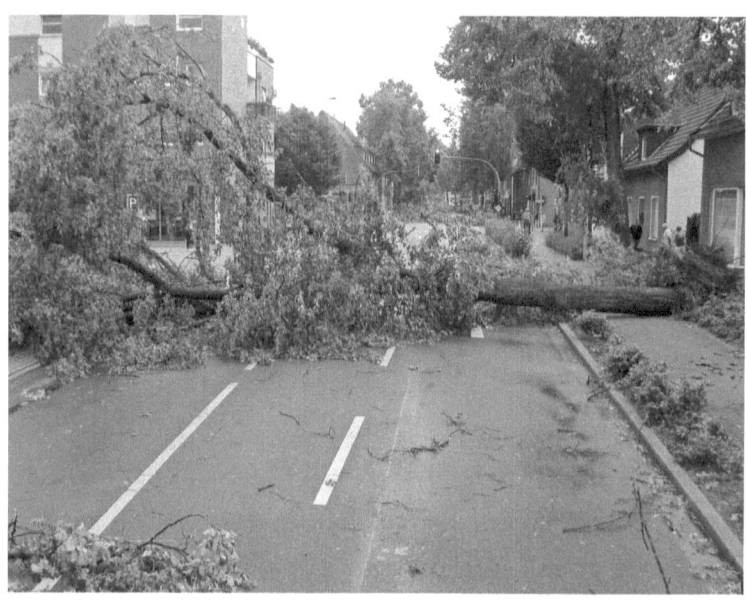

Think about all the wiring in that neighborhood immediately after the storm. At first it's down, then it comes up, little by little. Eventually people can turn on their lights without a brownout. And they can watch t.v., although it takes a while for them to get their heads on straight, after working around the clock to clean up their street.

That's what's going on in your system. You've got the t.v. on, but you keep hitting the wrong buttons on the remote, and the shows keep jumping around on your mental screen. It's just the recalibration process running its course, and until things get sorted, you're going to feel a little crazy.

But you're not going nuts. It just feels that way.

What to do?

Be patient with yourself. Your brain needs time to figure things out again.

Have a sense of humor. Seriously – some of the stuff you do is pretty funny, if you think about it. If your system is going to go haywire for a while, you might as well have fun with it. It's not the end of the world. Plus, you'll have a hell of a story to tell, on down the line.

9. You May Feel Like This For A While.

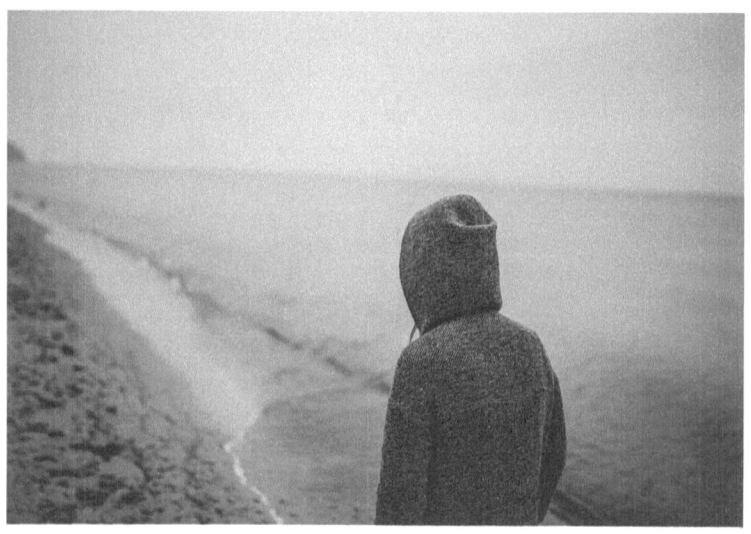

It feels like no one understands... and heck if you can describe it to them

Yep, it's unpleasant. Yep, it can suck. And yep, it can take a while to get all figured out.

It's practically impossible to explain to others what it feels like to have post-concussive symptoms, and it can be almost as impossible to convince other people that concussion / TBI is a thing. Heck, I have long-time friends and family who still refuse to believe I have any issues – and I'm not the only TBI survivor who has that experience.

Never mind that. Just take care of yourself and pay attention to your own recovery.

And don't lose hope. I had just about given up of ever feeling normal again, when suddenly I felt like my old self again.

It brought me to tears.

It was amazing.

And it comes and goes.

The thing to remember is that, through the course of life, we never ever stay the same person. We are constantly changing, constantly growing, and expecting ourselves to stay the way we were "before" isn't realistic.

It was never going to happen, anyway. Even if you hadn't gotten injured, life would have changed you in some way. You would have lost or gained many, many things (and people) along the way, and those experiences would have changed you, too.

Just be aware, that brain injury / concussion isn't the kind of thing you can rush. The brain will take its own sweet time.

So, buckle up for the ride of your life!

What to do?

The best thing you can do is be patient with yourself and be aware of the ways that you are not functioning as well as you would like. Make a note. Try again. And keep learning.

Don't rush it. These things take time. Eat healthy food, stay away from a lot of junk food, sugar, caffeine, and stress, drink plenty of water, and get lots of good sleep.

Exercise can also help a great deal. It reduces stress, and it gets your mind off your brain for a while. The times I've felt best, are the times I've been exercising regularly – even light exercise for 10 minutes at the start of each day. Just don't overdo it. Recovering from an injured brain is hassle enough, without adding an injured body to it.

10. Plenty Of Other People Have Had Concussions, And Most Of Them Are Getting On With Their Lives.

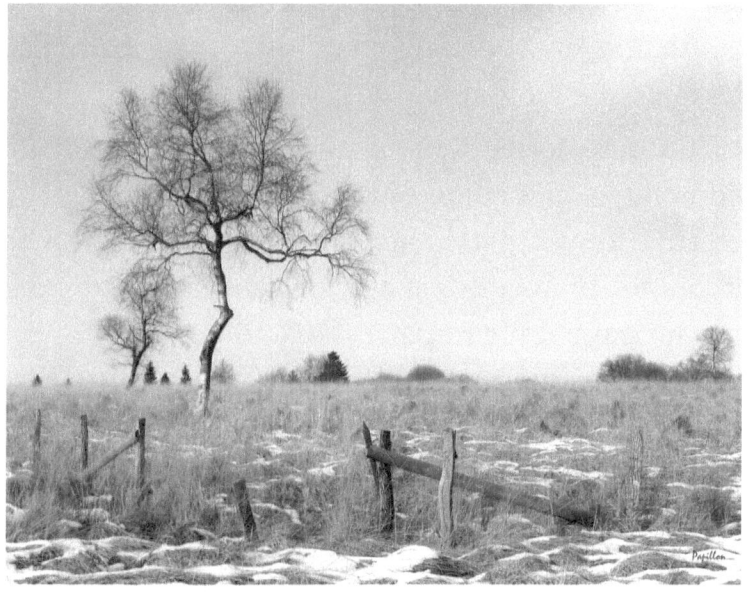

It's not the end. It may feel like it, but it's not

Brain injury / concussion is extremely common. Millions of people in the US experience one each year, and many more experience them globally.

Getting clunked on the head is something as old as the hills. If it were catastrophic every single time, the human race would not have survived. So take courage – you're in good company.

While brain injury recovery can be time-consuming and there are no hard-and-fast guarantees, rest assured that many people have bounced back after concussion and gone on to live productive, satisfying, fulfilling lives. Those who haven't had such an easy time are in the minority. And while I am a member of that minority, I can tell you that even the long, hard road has had many blessings along the way.

You may notice some changes in your personality and abilities, but some of the changes may be for the better. I know that in my case, overcoming all the difficulties of symptoms and blocks that were put in my way trained me to persevere and be diligent – and also to pay attention to important signals that I was screwing up again and needed to make a course correction.

Nobody wants to injure their brain. But when it happens, there's a lot of useful lessons to be learned. And those who learn and adapt, are the ones with the highest success rate.

You can be one of the successes. No doubt about it!

What to do?

Be patient.

Pay attention.

Be the best person you can.

Put forth your best effort and learn from all your mistakes.

And remember: This is not the end.

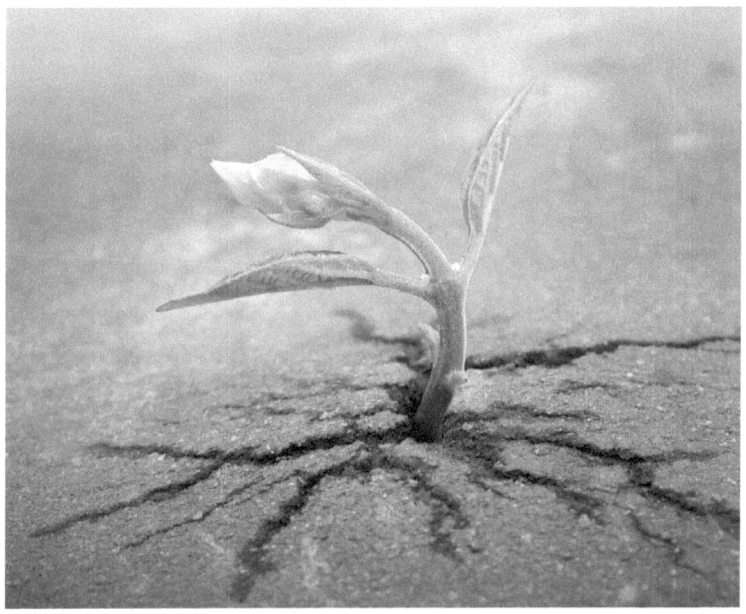

About the Author

BrokenBrilliant is a TBI blogger who shares their life experience with recovering from multiple mild traumatic brain injuries. Their blog can be found at **http://brokenbrilliant.wordpress.com**

www.ingramcontent.com/pod-product-compliance
Lightning Source LLC
Chambersburg PA
CBHW050338290526
45785CB00006B/2546